low carb Snacks

HEALTHY AND DELICIOUS
LOW CARB SNACK RECIPES
FOR EXTREME WEIGHT LOSS

Published by The Fruitful Mind
www.fruitfulbooks.com

Disclaimer

Table of Contents

Introduction

Cookies, granola bars, chips, ice cream, bagels and donuts are some of America's favourite snack foods but they are also loaded with sugar, fat and contain very little nutritional value. If you are trying to adhere to the low carb diet, finding healthy, wholesome snacks may pose a bit of a problem for you. The low carb snack recipes outlined in this cookbook all contain ingredients that have a low glycemic index so they won't spike your blood sugar levels; they also contain protein and some type of healthy fat.

Embracing the low-cab, ketogenic diet is one of the most beneficial ways to rejuvenate your health and drop those loathsome pounds. The recipes in this cookbook promote low carb digestion; they yield no more than ten net carbohydrates per serving, thus forcing your body into a sort of overdrive of weight loss. Low Carb Snacks is a cookbook designed to help you lose weight and take control of your life once more.

The low-carbohydrate diet is unrivalled, leaving its proponents with a slim-waist and six pack abs. But how, precisely, does it work? Let's look at the science. Essentially, carbohydrates are made up of glucose. Glucose is a sugar, and when it enters your body, it immediately lends itself to fueling your cells to do their everyday cell mechanisms. As you probably know, your cells are constantly working to keep you breathing, keep you moving, and keep you alive. And glucose is absolutely necessary in order to make that happen.

However, when you continually refuel yourself with glucose, your body has no need to look to other stored fat cells for fuel. Therefore, your body doesn't diminish its fat cell count; it continually works through the carbohydrates you fuel it with. You're making it easy on yourself, and you're doing your body no real favors. When you eat a low-carbohydrate diet, however, your body becomes confused. You are not lending it all the necessary glucose your cells require in order to work properly; therefore, your body must look to other sources. When you eat mostly fat and protein, the fat and protein have to undergo a process called ketosis. Your fat and protein molecules are transferred to glucose in the liver. Your body must work hard to do this, thus burning far more calories to digest these molecules than it usually does to digest foods rich in carbohydrates.

In addition, when you don't fuel yourself with a carbohydrate-stocked diet, you won't unnecessarily impact your blood sugar levels. After you eat a rich carbohydrate meal, your blood sugar spikes unnecessarily; this boosts your insulin levels. When your insulin and glucose levels fall once more, you're left craving sugary, carbohydrate-rich foods; the cycle will continue. However, when you regulate your carbohydrate intake, your body gets much better at regulating your appetite. Less carbohydrates means less insane sugar cravings.

This snack cookbook outlines 37 delicious, low carb snack recipes that are super easy to make and will effectively ease your hunger pains in between meals. Choose from tasty recipes such as the Spicy Mexican Lettuce Wraps, Vegan Stuffed Mushrooms, or Sweet Potato 'Nachos'. Lose weight, save time, and keep yourself well. Bring endless flavor into your life, and rejuvenate yourself. Food is the ultimate comfort, the ultimate fuel, and this cookbook eliminates its hassle once and for all!

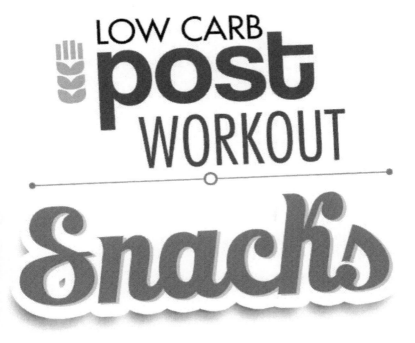

LOW CARB **post** WORKOUT Snacks

Barbecue Chicken Drumsticks

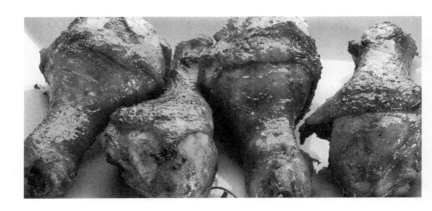

Making your own barbecue sauce ensures that it is low in sugars and this homemade version takes minimal preparation and cooking. This recipe can be used to marinade pork ribs, beef steaks or any other meat. Take a couple of protein packed drumsticks to the gym to give you a quick refill of energy after a workout session, a tasty enough reason to work out in the first place.

Serves: 4
Preparation time: 10 minutes, plus 1 hour marinating

Ingredients

1 medium white onion
2 cloves garlic
1 cup orange juice
2 tsp English mustard
2 tsp ground ginger
1 tsp mild/hot chilli powder
1 tbsp dried parsley
1 can chopped tomatoes, drained
8 chicken drumsticks

Method

1. Fine chop the onion and garlic.

2. Put everything except the chicken into a pan and bring to the boil, then simmer for 15 minutes, check for seasoning and add salt and black pepper to taste.

3. Score the skin on the chicken to allow the flavours to penetrate right into the meat and put it in to a plastic tub. Cover the meat in the barbecue marinade and chill for at least an hour.

4. Preheat the oven to 375 degrees F.

5. Roast for 35-40 minutes until the chicken is cooked through.

6. Keep chilled until required.

Nutritional Information
Per serving

Calories	343
Fat (g)	14.1
Sodium (mg)	190.8
Net Carbohydrates (g)	8.8
Sugars (g)	7.7
Protein (g)	43

Cottage Cheese Salad Plate

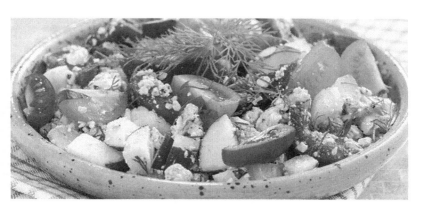

Cottage cheese is high in proteins which digest slowly, leaving you feeling fuller for longer. Any of these recipes are easily eaten on the go so ideal to take to the gym with you. Cottage cheese is also a great dip for low carb fruit and vegetables; you can also add your favourite herbs or spices to give it some extra flavour.

Serves: 4
Preparation time: 15 minutes

Ingredients
8 medium eggs

8 cherry tomatoes

1 red pepper

8 radishes

1 bunch of spring onions

2 cups cottage cheese

Method
1. Boil the eggs for 10 minutes, cool and remove the shells. Cut them into quarters and put 2 full eggs in each salad plate.

2. Chop all of the salad vegetables and add to the eggs.

3. Mix in the cottage cheese.

4. Season with salt and black pepper to taste.

5. Keep chilled until required.

Nutritional Information
Per serving

Calories	255
Fat (g)	11
Sodium (mg)	614

Net Carbohydrates (g)	9.3
Sugars (g)	7
Protein (g)	28

Scotch Eggs

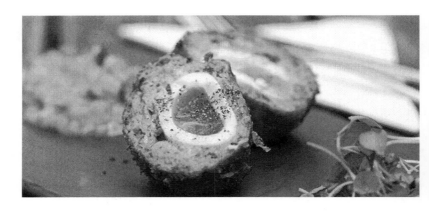

A traditional British picnic snack, these are easily portable and protein packed. Ensure you use high quality, non-processed sausage meat.

Serves: 4
Preparation time: 15 minutes

Ingredients
5 large eggs
1 pound pork sausage meat
1 cup parmesan cheese
Salt and pepper to taste

Method

1. Preheat the oven to 375 degrees F.

2. Boil 4 of the eggs for 10 minutes. Cool in cold water and peel off the shells.

3. Take a quarter of the meat and roll it out. Put the egg in the middle of it and tightly wrap the meat around it so it is a tight little ball.

4. Roll the meat covered eggs in the parmesan and a little black pepper.

5. Beat the remaining egg and brush it over the parmesan coating.

6. Cook for 25-35 minutes until golden brown.

7. Keep chilled until required.

Nutritional Information

Per serving

Calories	376
Fat (g)	23
Sodium (mg)	373
Net Carbohydrates (g)	7.5
Sugars (g)	2
Protein (g)	27

No Bake Protein Bars

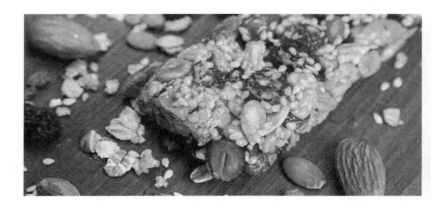

Protein bars have long been a post-workout staple to refuel the body. Choose your favourite from this selection of simple but effective recipes.

Makes: 6
Preparation time: 10 minutes

Ingredients
2 tbsp ground almonds
2 tbsp sesame seeds
12 tbsp protein powder
8 tbsp butter
2 tsp vanilla essence

Method

1. Mix all the dry ingredients in a bowl and season with a little salt and black pepper.

2. Melt the butter and add to the mix along with the vanilla.

3. Take ½ a cup of water and gradually add to the mixture until it is a soft and smooth dough and not sticky.

4. Grease and line a baking tin and pack the protein mixture in.

5. Chill overnight until set.

6. Store in an airtight container until required.

Nutritional Information

Per serving

Calories	472
Fat (g)	35
Sodium (mg)	168
Net Carbohydrates (g)	8.6
Sugars (g)	3
Protein (g)	28

Peanut Butter Protein Bars

Makes: 12
Preparation time: 5 minutes

Ingredients
1 cup chunky peanut butter
1 ½ cup almond meal
2 eggs whites
½ cup cashews
½ cup almonds

Method
1. Preheat the oven to 350 degrees F.
2. Thoroughly mix all the ingredients together.
3. Press the mixture into a lined baking dish and bake for 15 minutes.
4. Cool in the tin then cut into individual bars.
5. Keep chilled until required.

Nutritional Information

Per serving

Calories	172
Fat (g)	14
Sodium (mg)	9
Net carbohydrates (g)	3
Sugars (g)	1
Protein (g)	7

Nutty Banana Protein Bars

Makes: 8
Preparation time: 15 minutes

Ingredients
3 oz. protein powder
½ tsp salt
2 tablespoons almond flour
1 very ripe banana
5 tablespoons peanut butter
½ tbsp coconut oil
½ cup old fashioned rolled oats
1 tbsp almonds
1 tbsp raisins

Method
1. Preheat the oven to 350 degrees F.

2. Mix together the protein powder, salt and flour.

3. Mash the banana and add it to the dry ingredients along with the peanut butter and oil. Continue to mash it all until well combined.

4. Add the oats and mix the hard dough as well as possible. Stir the almonds and raisins in.

5. Bake for 20 minutes. Cool in the tin then cut into individual bars.

6. Freeze overnight.

7. Keep chilled until required.

Nutritional Information
Per serving

Calories	128
Fat (g)	5
Sodium (mg)	83
Net carbohydrates (g)	10
Sugars (g)	4
Protein (g)	9

Kale Chips

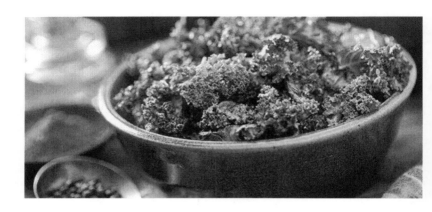

These are fantastic to have on the table for friends to nibble on during a relaxed get together. Or divide a batch into sealable plastic bags to eat on the go at any time.

Serves: 8
Preparation time: 10 minutes

Ingredients
A bunch of kale (curly is best for this recipe)
4 tbsp olive oil
2 tsp salt
½ tsp black pepper

Method

1. Preheat the oven to 350 degrees F.

2. Cut the stems off the kale leaves and tear into small pieces.

3. Wash the leaves and dry them as thoroughly as possible.

4. Toss the chips in a bowl with the oil, salt and pepper.

5. Bake for 10-15 minutes until beginning to brown.

6. Store in an airtight container until required.

Nutritional Information

Per serving

Calories	33
Fat (g)	0.5
Sodium (mg)	25
Net carbohydrates (g)	6
Sugars (g)	0
Protein (g)	2.9

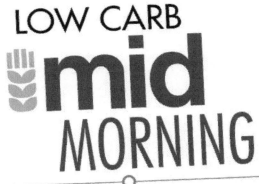

LOW CARB
mid
MORNING

Snacks

Bacon and Feta Mini Frittatas

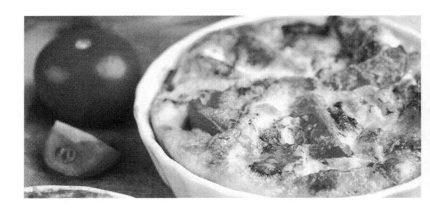

Ideal for breakfast on the go. Make a batch at the start of the week and just grab a couple from the fridge whenever you need a quick snack.

Makes 12
Preparation time: 15 minutes

Ingredients
6 rashers of smoked bacon
1 small white onion
1 tbsp olive oil
A large handful of spinach
3.5 oz. feta cheese
6 medium eggs

100ml 2% milk

Method

1. Preheat the oven to 350 degrees F.

2. Finely chop the bacon and onion then fry gently in the oil for 5-8 minutes until the bacon is coloured and the onion soft. Add the spinach to wilt down for 2 minutes.

3. Crumble the feta into the pan and stir everything together then season with some salt and black pepper.

4. Grease a 12 hole muffin tin with a little oil then share out the bacon filling evenly between the holes.

5. Whisk together the eggs and milk and season well. Pour the eggs over the filling.

6. Bake for 20-25 minutes, until golden brown and set.

7. Keep chilled until required.

Nutritional Information
Per frittata

Calories	182
Fat (g)	12.7
Sodium (mg)	74.2
Net carbohydrates (g)	3.1
Sugars (g)	1.4
Protein (g)	14.2

Breakfast Hash

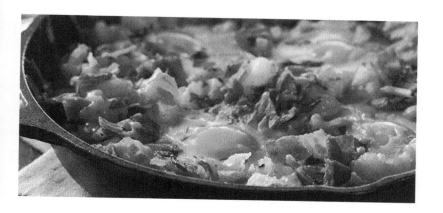

A filling snack that packs you with energy for the day ahead, especially helpful on hungover weekend mornings.

Serves: 4
Preparation time: 25 minutes

Ingredients
1 lb. cauliflower
1 medium white onion
2 tbsp olive oil
8 cherry tomatoes
8 mushrooms
4 rashers smoked bacon
2 sausages

1 tbsp chopped parsley

4 medium eggs

Method

1. Grate the cauliflower so it resembles breadcrumbs and chop the onion.

2. Heat the oil in a large frying pan and fry the cauliflower and onion for 15 minutes until brown and crisp, stir regularly.

3. Preheat the boiler to high.

4. Slice the tomatoes and mushrooms into quarters. Roughly cut the meat into evenly sized chunks and add to the pan for 10 minutes along with salt and black pepper, continue stirring. Stir in the parsley.

5. Make 4 wells, near each corner, and break an egg into each one.

6. Place under the preheated boiler for 5-10 minutes until the eggs have set.

7. Serve while hot.

Nutritional Information

Per serving

Calories	168
Fat (g)	11.1
Sodium (mg)	578.4
Carbohydrates (g)	7.5
Sugars (g)	2.6
Protein (g)	10.6

Blueberry Pancakes with Bacon

These American style pancakes are perfect for a weekend treat and only take a few minutes to prepare and cook.

Serves: 6
Preparation time: 5 minutes

Ingredients
12 rashers smoked bacon
¾ cups almond flour
1 egg
300ml 2% milk
1 tsp baking powder
1 tsp salt
½ cup blueberries
Olive oil

Method
1. Whisk together the flour, egg, milk, baking powder and salt.
2. Stir the blueberries into the batter.
3. Fry the bacon for 3-5 minutes each side depending on taste, turn halfway through cooking.

4. Heat a little olive oil in a frying pan and cook the pancakes in batches of 4 for 2-3 minutes on each side until both are golden brown.

5. Serve the pancakes topped with the bacon immediately.

Nutritional Information

Per serving

Calories	340
Fat (g)	24.1
Sodium (mg)	1236
Net carbohydrates (g)	9.8
Sugars (g)	5.6
Protein (g)	22.8

Almond Milk Green Smoothie

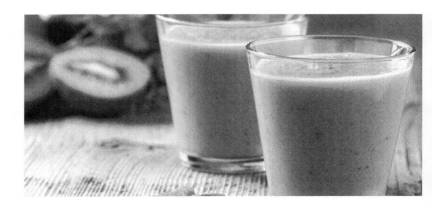

Almond milk is very low in carbs and is lactose free. It also contains no cholesterol or saturated fat so is an excellent choice for those suffering from heart conditions.

Serves: 1
Preparation time: 5 minutes

Ingredients
1 stick celery
1 cup kale (washed and de-stemmed)
½ kiwi
1 cup almond milk

Method

1. Roughly chop all the fruit and vegetables and blend with the milk until smooth.

2. Serve immediately or keep chilled until required.

Nutritional Information

Per serving

Calories	73
Fat (g)	3
Sodium (mg)	185
Net carbohydrates (g)	9
Sugars (g)	4
Protein (g)	3

Berry Smoothie

Serves: 1
Preparation time: 5 minutes

Ingredients
¼ cup blackberries
¼ cup blueberries
Handful spinach
250ml almond milk
2 tsp vanilla essence

Method
1. Blend all ingredients together.
2. Serve immediately for keep chilled until required.

Nutritional Information
Per serving

Calories	110
Fat (g)	5
Sodium (mg)	368
Net carbohydrates (g)	9
Sugars (g)	6
Protein (g)	4

Greek Yogurt with Walnut and Flax Seed

If you like a bit of crunch in a morning then use this recipe to make your own low carb snack cereal using seeds and nuts.

Serves: 4
Preparation time: 5 minutes

Ingredients
½ cup raspberries
2 cups Greek yogurt (plain)
4 tbsp chopped walnuts
4 tbsp flax seeds
1 tsp vanilla extract

Method
1. Roughly chop the raspberries.
2. Mix together all the ingredients.
3. Serve immediately or keep chilled until required.

Nutritional Information

Per serving

Calories	256
Fat (g)	17
Sodium (mg)	53
Net carbohydrates (g)	9
Sugars (g)	6
Protein (g)	17

Coconut Flour Egg Bread

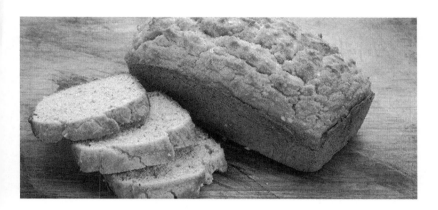

A quick and easy bread to make as it doesn't require long kneading time. Coconut flour is high in protein as well as being gluten free.

Serves: 4
Preparation time: 5 minutes

Ingredients
½ tsp cider vinegar
½ tsp baking soda
½ cup coconut flour
1 medium egg
6 medium egg whites
2 tsp vanilla extract

¼ tsp salt.
8 medium eggs
Olive oil

Method
1. Preheat the oven to 350 degrees F.
2. Mix the vinegar and baking soda in a small bowl.
3. Put all the other ingredients in a large bowl and combine. Add the vinegar mix and stir as it begins to bubble.
4. Pour the mixture into a greased loaf tin.
5. Bake for 45-50 minutes until light brown.
6. Beat the eggs in a flat dish and season well with salt and black pepper.
7. Slice the loaf.
8. Heat a little oil in a frying pan. Dip the bread into the eggs until coated then fry on high for 3-4 minutes on each side until both are golden brown.
9. Serve while hot.

Nutritional Information
Per serving

Calories	235
Fat (g)	12
Sodium (mg)	565
Carbohydrates (g)	9
Sugars (g)	2
Protein (g)	20

High Protein Almond Muffins

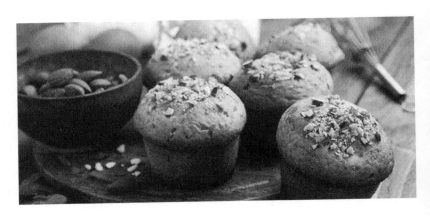

Avoid extra sugar and carbs by using apple juice and ground almonds so you can still enjoy breakfast muffins on the go.

Makes 12
Preparation time: 10 minutes

Ingredients
2 cups almond meal
5 scoops vanilla protein powder
1tbsp cinnamon
1 tsp nutmeg
4 tbsp butter
4 medium eggs

1 cup apple juice

Method

1. Preheat the oven to 350 degrees F.
2. Place all the dry ingredients into a bowl then knead the butter in.
3. Beat the eggs and fold in along with the juice. Mix until thoroughly combined.
4. Spoon the mixture into muffin tins to about ¾ full and bake for 10-15 minutes until just browned.
5. Store in an airtight container until required.

Nutritional Information
Per serving

Calories	244
Fat (g)	17
Sodium (mg)	196
Net carbohydrates (g)	7
Sugars (g)	4
Protein (g)	15

LOW CARB midday

Snacks

Roasted Mediterranean Vegetable Frittata

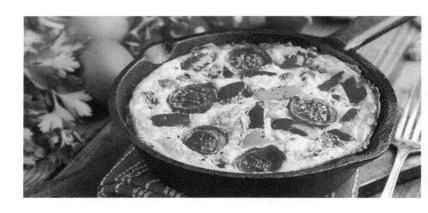

This traditional Italian omelette is packed full of Mediterranean flavours and vegetables. Cut it into wedges and eat it cold. It is also suitable for vegetarians and gluten free.

Serves: 4
Preparation time: 15 minutes

Ingredients
1 red onion
1 small courgette
1 orange pepper
½ aubergine

8 cherry tomatoes

6 mushrooms

10 black olives

2 tbsp olive oil

Handful of fresh basil

6 medium eggs

1/3 cup 2% milk

¼ cup Parmesan cheese

1/3 cup mozzarella cheese

Method

1. Preheat the oven to 400 degrees F.

2. Thickly chop the onion, courgette, pepper and aubergine into evenly sized, chunky pieces. Cut the tomatoes, mushrooms and olives in half.

3. Mix all the vegetables together in a large roasting tray and drizzle with the oil.

4. Roast for 40 minutes, until soft but not mushy.

5. Roughly chop the basil and add to the vegetables while they are still warm.

6. Finely grate the parmesan and tear the mozzarella into small pieces.

7. Whisk the eggs and milk together in a large bowl and season well with salt and black pepper.

8. Add the roasted vegetables and cheeses to the eggs and mix well.

9. Preheat the broiler to high.

10. Heat the oil in a large, oven proof frying pan and pour the frittata mix. Cook for 5-10 minutes until it's beginning to set, stirring occasionally.

11. Put the frittata under the broiler for a further 5-10 minutes until it's fully set.

12. Cool in the pan then cut into wedges and chill until required.

Nutritional Information

Per serving:

Calories	221
Fat (g)	13.9
Sodium (mg)	280
Net carbohydrates (g)	8.7
Sugars (g)	4.5
Protein (g)	17.3

Marinated Monkfish and Prawn Kebabs

These light kebabs are ideal to add to your summer barbecue menu but can also be cooked under a hot grill at any time of the year.

Serves: 4
Preparation time: 15 minutes plus 1 hour marinating

Ingredients
½ pound monkfish steak
20 tiger prawns
2 cloves garlic
2 tbsp olive oil
Juice of a lime
2cm freshly grated ginger root
2 tsp cayenne pepper
20 cherry tomatoes

Method
1. Cut the monkfish into chunks a similar size to the prawns and put them into a plastic tub.

2. Put the garlic, oil, lime juice, ginger and pepper into a blender along with some salt and black pepper and blend until well mixed then pour it over the fish and prawns.

3. Cover the tub and chill for at least an hour.

4. Thread the fish, prawns and tomatoes onto kebab skewers and cook on the hottest part of the barbecue for 3-5 minutes on each side until pink and cooked through. Alternatively, you can broil in the over on high.

5. Serve while hot.

Nutritional Information

Per serving

Calories	178
Fat (g)	1.2
Sodium (mg)	180.6
Net carbohydrates (g)	6.5
Sugars (g)	2.4
Protein (g)	37.3

Aubergines Stuffed with Moussaka

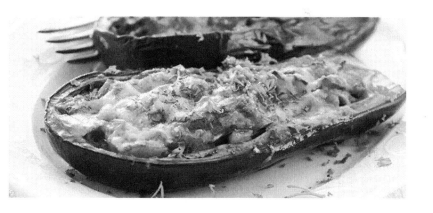

A new way to serve moussaka that can be packed into lunchboxes for a healthy and tasty midday treat.

Serves: 4
Preparation time: 30 minutes

Ingredients
2 large aubergines
1 medium onion
1 garlic clove
1 tbsp olive oil
½ pound ground lamb (you can substitute another ground meat)

¼ cup red wine

1 tin chopped tomatoes, drained

2 tsp dried oregano

2 tsp ground cinnamon

¼ cup ricotta cheese

¼ cup Parmesan cheese

1 tsp ground nutmeg

Method

1. Preheat the oven to 425 degrees F.

2. Scoop the insides out of the aubergines and keep it for filling. Coat them in a little oil and place on a baking tray.

3. Dice the onion and garlic.

4. Heat the oil and fry the onion and garlic for 3-4 minutes on medium heat until they begin to soften then add the lamb for 10-15 minutes until fully browned.

5. Add the wine and bring to a boil for 2 minutes, reduce heat down to a simmer.

6. Add the tomatoes, oregano, cinnamon and retained aubergine insides to the pan for 5 minutes then season with salt and black pepper.

7. In a bowl, mash together the ricotta, parmesan and nutmeg.

8. Fill the aubergines with the meat then top with the cheese mixture.

9. Bake for 5-10 minutes until the cheese has melted and is starting to brown.

10. Serve immediately or chill until required.

Nutritional Information
Per serving

Calories	376
Fat (g)	23.4
Sodium (mg)	252.5
Net carbohydrates (g)	10
Sugars (g)	7.7
Protein (g)	26

Spicy Mexican Lettuce Wraps

Try a Mexican classic wrapped in a low carb alternative.

Serves: 4
Preparation time: 25 minutes

Ingredients
2 chicken breasts
1 medium white onion
1 red pepper
2 tbsp olive oil
Mild or hot chilli powder
¼ cup cheddar cheese
1 avocado
4 large lettuce leaves
Sour cream

Method
1. Dice the chicken, onion and pepper.
2. Heat the oil in a frying pan and cook the chicken, onion, pepper and chilli powder on high for 10-15 minutes until the chicken is cooked through, season with a little salt and black pepper.

3. Grate the cheese and slice the avocado.

4. Divide the chicken mix between the leaves, top with the cheese, avocado slices and a spoonful of sour cream. Grind over some black pepper.

5. Serve immediately or chill until required.

Nutritional Information

Per serving

Calories	233
Fat (g)	16.2
Sodium (mg)	189.9
Net carbohydrates (g)	5.4
Sugars (g)	1.2
Protein (g)	15.2

Burgers in Mushroom Buns

Following a low carb diet doesn't mean missing out on everyday meals. These super tasty buns mean you won't even notice the lack of bread.

Serves: 4
Preparation time: 5 minutes

Ingredients
1 medium white onion
1 lb. lean ground beef
2 tsp paprika
8 Portobello mushrooms
½ cup cheddar cheese

Method
1. Preheat the grill to medium.
2. Fine chop the onion and mix thoroughly into the meat along with the paprika and some salt and black pepper. Shape into 4 evenly sized burgers.
3. Clean out the inside of the mushrooms then rub some olive oil all over them.

4. Grill the mushrooms and burgers for 5-8 minutes each side until the burgers are cooked through.

5. Put a sprinkling of cheese on each burger 2 minutes before the end of cooking to melt.

6. Build the burgers with one mushroom on the bottom followed by the meat. Secure the other mushroom on the top with cocktail sticks.

7. Serve while hot.

Nutritional Information

Per serving

Calories	344
Fat (g)	14.2
Sodium (mg)	204.1
Net carbohydrates (g)	9.2
Sugars (g)	5.3
Protein (g)	40.4

Spanakopita Cups with Sesame Seed Crumble

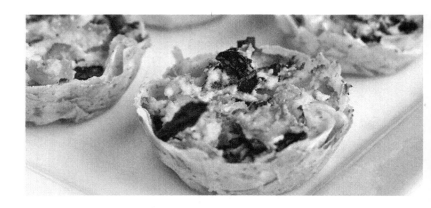

Serves: 4
Preparation time: 15 minutes

Ingredients
1 bag of spinach
1 bunch of spring onions
2 tsp olive oil
½ cup feta
1 egg
2 tsp chopped dill
1 tsp ground nutmeg
Zest of 1 lemon
2 tbsp sesame seeds
Lettuce leaves

Method

1. Preheat the oven to 375 degrees F.

2. Wash the spinach then put in a sauce pan and cover. Cook for 4-5 minutes until wilted down, stirring occasionally.

3. Chop the onions and cut the feta into squares. Beat the egg.

4. Drain the spinach then dry as thoroughly as possible on kitchen paper.

5. Heat the oil in the spinach pan and soften the onions for 4-5 minutes. Add all the other ingredients, season well with black pepper and stir until fully combined.

6. Bake for 30 minutes until golden brown.

7. Toast the sesame seeds for 3-5 minutes in a dry frying pan until slightly darkened.

7. Wrap the filling in a lettuce leaf, sprinkle over the toasted seeds and secure with a cocktail stick.

8. Serve immediately or chill until required.

Nutritional Information

Per serving

Calories	210
Fat (g)	14.5
Sodium (mg)	104.8
Net carbohydrates (g)	7
Sugars (g)	0
Protein (g)	13.9

Chorizo Stuffed Peppers

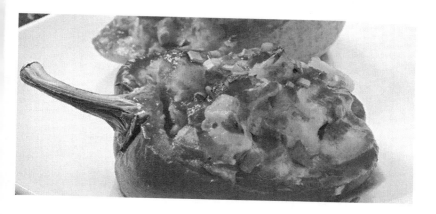

These stuffed peppers can be eaten like a sandwich at any time. Save the leftover homemade pesto to add to any recipe to give it an extra injection of low carb flavour.

Serves: 4
Preparation time: 15 minutes

Ingredients
Large handful of basil
¼ cup parmesan cheese
2 garlic cloves
150ml olive oil

150g chorizo
1 medium onion
¾ cup cheddar cheese
1 tbsp olive oil
2 sweet peppers

Method

1. Preheat the oven to 375 degrees F.

2. Rough chop the basil, finely grate the parmesan, finely chop the garlic and put them all in a food processor. Blend with the olive oil until smooth then keep chilled.

3. Cut the chorizo into small chunks, finely dice the onion and grate the cheddar cheese.

4. Heat the olive oil, in a frying pan and cook the onion for 3-4 minutes until soft.

5. Mix the onion, chorizo and cheese together in a bowl.

6. Cut the peppers in half and rub with the tbsp of oil. Place them open side up on a baking tray and share out the chorizo and cheese filling between them.

7. Bake for 15-20 minutes until heated through and cheese is melted and beginning to brown.

8. Serve them immediately, drizzled with a little of the pesto or chill until required.

Nutritional Information
Per serving

Calories	415
Fat (g)	34
Sodium (mg)	772
Net carbohydrates (g)	5
Sugars (g)	4
Protein (g)	20

Cauliflower Hash Browns

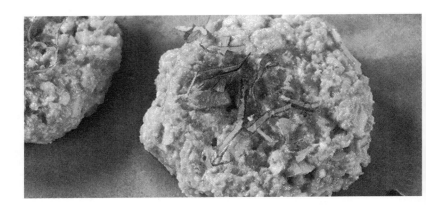

As satisfying as traditional carb filled hash browns, this cauliflower version is as healthy as it is delicious.

Serves: 4
Preparation time: 10 minutes

Ingredients
1 lb. cauliflower crowns
1 medium onion
1 medium egg
Olive oil

Method

1. Grate the cauliflower and finely dice the onion.

2. Mix everything together and add the egg.

3. Heat the oil in a frying pan and cook tablespoons of the mixture for 2-3 minutes on each side until crispy and brown.

4. Serve while hot.

Nutritional Information

Per serving

Calories	160
Fat (g)	10
Sodium (mg)	233
Net carbohydrates (g)	10
Sugars (g)	4
Protein (g)	8

Broccoli Cheese

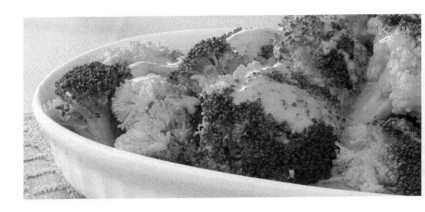

Broccoli contains more protein, iron and vitamins A, K and C than cauliflower so try out this classic vegetable dish with a twist.

Serves: 4
Preparation time: 15 minutes

Ingredients
4 cups broccoli
4 tbsp butter
60g almond flour
500ml almond milk
2 tsp wholegrain mustard
450g gruyere cheese

Method

1. Preheat the oven to 350 degrees F.

2. Cut the broccoli into florets.

3. Cook the broccoli for 4 minutes in boiling water and drain.

4. Melt the butter in a large saucepan then stir in the flour to a smooth paste.

5. Gradually whisk in the milk, 100ml at a time, ensuring the sauce remains lump free.

6. Whisk in the mustard and a little salt and black pepper.

7. Stir the cheese in and mix until it is fully melted.

8. Mix the broccoli into the cheese sauce until it's completely covered then transfer it all into a roasting dish.

9. Bake for 20-25 minutes until bubbling and beginning to brown.

10. Serve while hot.

Nutritional Information

Per serving

Calories	659
Fat (g)	54
Sodium (mg)	1044
Net carbohydrates (g)	8
Sugars (g)	2
Protein (g)	38

Radish Chips

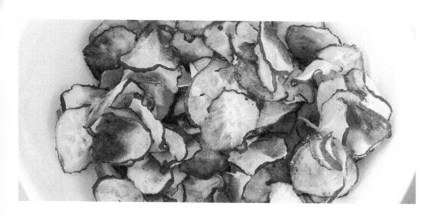

This is easily the tastiest way to eat radish. Make a big batch up and bag individual portions so you can throw one in your bag to snack on during the day.

Serves: 4
Preparation time: 15 minutes

Ingredients
80 radishes
Olive oil
Salt and pepper

Method

1. Preheat the oven to 400 degrees F.

2. Thinly slice the radishes then toss in enough oil to coat them.

3. Season well with salt and black pepper. (At this point you can also add any herbs or spices you wish too)

4. Cook for 10 minutes then turn them over. Cook for a further 5-15 minutes until crisp and golden brown. Check often during the second cooking time as they can quickly burn.

5. Store in an airtight container until required.

Nutritional Information

Per serving

Calories	6
Fat (g)	0
Sodium (mg)	16
Net carbohydrates (g)	1
Sugars (g)	1
Protein (g)	0

Hot Dogs and Coleslaw

Hotdogs without the bun cuts out most of the carbs from this dish and making your own coleslaw ensures the vegetable sugars are kept low.

Serves: 4
Preparation time: 15 minutes

Ingredients
8 good quality sausages
½ small white cabbage
2 medium sized carrots
½ red onion
3 tbsp mayonnaise
1 tbsp parsley

Method
1. Grill the sausages under a hot grill for 15-20 minutes, turning every 5 minutes, until browned all over and cooked through.
2. Finely shred the cabbage, grate the carrots then finely slice the onion.

3. Mix all the ingredients together, season with salt and black pepper and serve with the hot sausages.
4. Keep any leftover coleslaw chilled until required.

Nutritional Information
Per serving

Calories	255
Fat (g)	20
Sodium (mg)	478
Net carbohydrates (g)	9
Sugars (g)	5
Protein (g)	10

Smoked Mackerel Mousse with Baby Corn

A super simple recipe that can be made in minutes, also good as a dinner party starter. You can substitute the corn for any lower carb crudité if you choose or eat it on the cheesy cracker recipe further on in this book.

Serves: 2
Preparation time: 5 minutes

Ingredients
Approx. 8 baby corn ears
250g smoked mackerel
1 tsp freshly grated horseradish
2 tbsp crème fraîche
¼ lemon juice
7 tbsp butter

Method
1. Blanch the baby corn for 2 minutes in boiling water.
2. Blend all the other ingredients together until smooth.

3. Serve the corn and mousse immediately or chill until required.

Nutritional Information

Per serving

Calories	493
Fat (g)	52
Sodium (mg)	617
Net carbohydrates (g)	10
Sugars (g)	2
Protein (g)	8

LOW CARB evening

Snacks

Parmesan Onion Rings

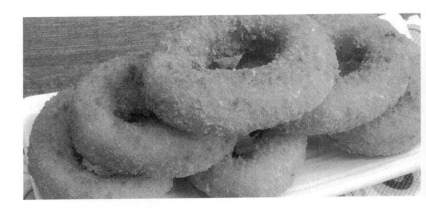

Coating your onion rings in low carb flour ensures you don't have to miss out on your favourite evening treats. Great for serving up to the gang for the big game.

Serves: 4
Preparation time: 10 minutes

Ingredients
Vegetable oil, for deep frying
1 large white onion
1 tbsp parmesan cheese
1 tbsp coconut flour
1 medium egg
1 tbsp heavy cream

Method

1. Heat the oil in a large pot to 350 degrees F.

2. Thickly slice the onion into rings.

3. Mix the cheese and flour together and season well with black pepper.

4. Beat the egg and cream together.

5. Dip the onion rings first into the wet mixture, then the dry and carefully put into the hot oil.

6. Fry for 2-3 minutes until golden brown and drain on kitchen paper before serving while hot.

Nutritional Information

Per serving

Calories	89
Fat (g)	7
Sodium (mg)	47
Net carbohydrates (g)	5
Sugars (g)	2
Protein (g)	3

Meatball, Sweet Potato and Shallot Kebabs

Southern inspired pork meatballs and low carb but tasty vegetables make for a delicious evening nibble, whether cooked on the barbecue or the grill.

Serves: 4
Preparation time: 10 minutes

Ingredients
1 medium sweet potato
1 tbsp coriander
2 tsp cayenne pepper
450g ground pork
8 shallots

Method
1. Peel the sweet potato and cut it into medium sized chunks. Microwave on high for 2-4 minutes until soft enough to put onto skewers.
2. Mix the coriander, cayenne and pork together with your hands and season well with salt and black pepper. Shape into 16-20 meatballs.

3. Thread the potato chunks, meatballs and shallots onto kebab sticks and drizzle with olive oil.

4. Broil or barbecue on medium high for 15-20 minutes until the meat is cooked through and the vegetables are browning.

5. Serve immediately while hot.

Nutritional Information
Per serving

Calories	200
Fat (g)	9
Sodium (mg)	82
Net carbohydrates (g)	9.6
Sugars (g)	4
Protein (g)	24

Sweet Potato 'Nachos'

Comforting carbs are still on option as long as you choose options such as sweet potatoes. You can add herbs, spices or garlic to the oil to add different flavours to your nachos.

Serves: 4-6
Preparation time: 10 minutes

Ingredients
3 large sweet potatoes
2 tbsp olive oil
Salt and pepper

Method
1. Preheat the oven to 375 degrees F.
2. Peel the potatoes and slice them very thinly. Toss them in the oil and season very well with salt and black pepper.
3. Bake for 10 minutes on each side, removing them as they begin to turn brown.
4. Serve while still warm or store in an airtight container and chill until required.

Nutritional Information

Per serving

Calories	71
Fat (g)	4
Sodium (mg)	605
Net carbohydrates (g)	9
Sugars (g)	3
Protein (g)	1

Vegan Stuffed Mushrooms

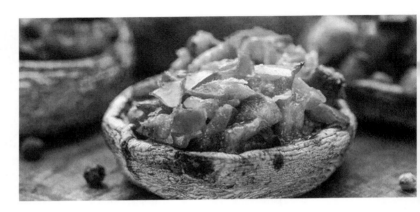

This vegan low carb snack can be made with regular cheese, or cottage cheese, if you prefer.

Serves: 4
Preparation time: 30 minutes

Ingredients
⅓ cup quinoa
4 portobello mushrooms
1 tbsp butter
100g leeks
½ cup vegan parmesan cheese
1 tbsp dill

Method

1. Preheat the oven to 350 degrees F.

2. Simmer the quinoa in 2/3 cup of water for 15 minutes, until most of the liquid has been absorbed. Remove from heat and put to one side, covered.

3. Rub the mushrooms in a little olive oil and bake for 10 minutes, empty.

4. Melt the butter in a small pan, slice the leeks and cook on medium for 5-10 minutes until soft but not coloured.

5. Finely grate the cheese.

6. Mix together the leeks, ¼ cup of the cheese and dill, season with salt and black pepper and spoon it into the hot mushrooms.

7. Sprinkle the rest of the cheese over the top and return to the oven for 10-15 minutes until the cheese is beginning to brown.

8. Serve immediately or chill until required.

Nutritional Information
Per serving

Calories	104
Fat (g)	5
Sodium (mg)	116
Net carbohydrates (g)	10
Sugars (g)	2
Protein (g)	6

Oopsie Rolls

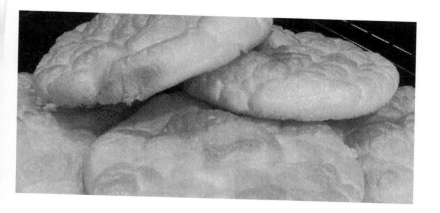

An oopsie roll is similar to a bread bun although carb, and gluten, free. Make a big batch at the start of the week so you can quickly make an open sandwich any time you feel hungry. Perfect for a light snack at the end of the day or for lunch.

Makes: 6 rolls
Preparation time: 10 minutes

Ingredients
3 eggs
Pinch of cream of tartar
100g (3oz.) cream cheese

Method

1. Preheat the oven to 300 degrees F.

2. Separate all the eggs, putting the whites in one bowl and the yolks in another.

3. Ensure the egg white bowl is scrupulously clean or the whites won't stiffen properly.

4. Add the cream of tartare to the egg whites and whisk into stiff peaks.

5. Add the cheese and a pinch of salt to the yolks and whisk until combined and smooth.

6. Gently fold the whites into the yolks trying to keep as much air in them as possible.

7. Spoon the mixture into six large mounds onto a greased and lined baking tray and cook for 30-40 minutes until golden brown but not crumbly.

Store in an airtight container until required.

Nutritional Information
Per serving

Calories	64
Fat (g)	6.6
Sodium (mg)	85
Net carbohydrates (g)	1.7
Sugars (g)	0.6
Protein (g)	3.6

Smoked Salmon 'Bruschetta'

Serves: 6
Preparation time: 5 minutes

Ingredients
6 oopsie rolls
300g cream cheese
150g smoked salmon
½ cucumber

Method
1. Slice the oopsie rolls in half through the middle and spread evenly with the cream cheese.
2. Top each roll with a little of the salmon and a couple of cucumber slices. Grind over some black pepper.
3. Serve immediately.

Nutritional Information
Per serving

Calories	242
Fat (g)	20.9
Sodium (mg)	413

Net carbohydrates (g)	5.6
Sugars (g)	3.9
Protein (g)	12.9

Peach and Basil Oopsie Roll 'Bruschetta'

A delicious vegetarian dessert style sandwich.

Serves: 6
Preparation time: 5 minutes

Ingredients
6 oopsie rolls
300g cream cheese
Large handful of fresh basil
3 peaches

Method
1. Roughly chop the basil.
2. Cut the peaches into wedges.
3. Slice the oopsie rolls in half through the middle and spread evenly with the cream cheese.
4. Top each roll with a little basil and peach wedges. Grind over some black pepper.
5. Serve immediately.

Nutritional Information
Per serving

Calories	85
Fat (g)	6.8
Sodium (mg)	86.8
Net carbohydrates (g)	6.7
Sugars (g)	4.6
Protein (g)	4.1

Chicken and Celery Soup

Perfect to sip on a cold winter's evening, especially if you're feeling under the weather. The celery adds flavour to this soup and also adds low carb bulk to fill you up.

Serves: 4
Preparation time: 15 minutes

Ingredients
1 medium onion
2 cloves garlic
2 sticks celery
2 tbsp olive oil
350g chicken breast
1.5 litre chicken stock
2 tbsp cornflour
1 tbsp fresh parsley
1 tbsp cider vinegar

Method
1. Finely chop the onion, garlic and celery. Cut the chicken into medium sized pieces.

2. Melt the oil in a pan and cook the chicken, onion, garlic and celery for 5 minutes on a medium heat until softened but not coloured, stirring often.

3. Mix a little of the stock with the cornflour to make a smooth paste. Turn the heat up to high. Add the paste to the pan until dissolved, then add the rest of the stock.

4. Bring to a boil then simmer for 20 minutes.

5. Remove from the heat and stir through the parsley and vinegar, check for seasoning and add salt and black pepper to taste.

6. Serve while hot.

Nutritional Information

Per serving

Calories	238
Fat (g)	14
Sodium (mg)	82.6
Net carbohydrates (g)	5.6
Sugars (g)	0.8
Protein (g)	41

Pizza with a Cauliflower Crust

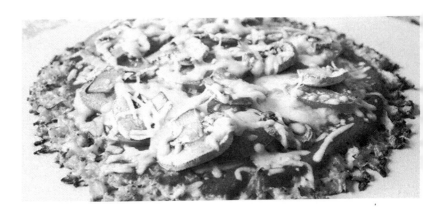

This twist on a traditional pizza crust keeps the carb count low and adds a new dimension of flavour to an old classic.

Serves: 4
Preparation time: 15 minutes

Ingredients
1 medium head of cauliflower
1 egg
1/3 cup parmesan cheese
¼ cup mozzarella cheese
¾ cup button mushrooms
¾ cup sliced ham
½ cup cheddar cheese

Method

1. Preheat the oven to 400 degrees F.

2. Cut the cauliflower into chunks and use a food processor to turn it into a fine breadcrumb texture.

3. Microwave it for 4-5 minutes until soft.

4. Beat the egg and stir it into the cauliflower then add the parmesan and mozzarella. **5.** Knead until it is a smooth dough.

6. Shape the dough into a round and flatten down.

7. Slice the mushrooms and tear the ham into small chunks.

8. Sprinkle the cheese over the pizza base then top with the mushrooms and ham.

9. Bake for 15-20 minutes until the base is firm and its edges are brown.

10. Serve while hot or keep chilled until required.

Nutritional Information

Per serving

Calories	388
Fat (g)	23.5
Sodium (mg)	1076
Net carbohydrates (g)	9.7
Sugars (g)	4.6
Protein (g)	37.4

10 Min Oriental Stir Fry

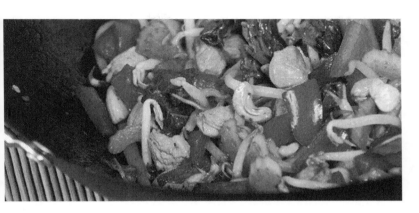

Serves: 1
Preparation time: 10 minutes

Ingredients
150g turkey breast
Olive oil
2oz mushrooms
2oz broccoli florets
2oz bean sprouts
2oz spinach
1 tsp 5 spice powder
1 tsp sesame oil

Method

1. Thin slice the turkey and slice the mushrooms.

2. Heat the olive oil in a wok and cook the turkey and mushrooms for 5 minutes, stirring regularly.

3. Add the broccoli and 5 spice powder to the wok for a further 5 minutes, season with salt and black pepper.

4. Add the spinach and when it has begun to wilt down, add the bean sprouts and the sesame oil.

5. Serve while hot.

Nutritional Information

Per serving

Calories	373
Fat (g)	22
Sodium (mg)	218
Net carbohydrates (g)	9
Sugars (g)	3
Protein (g)	39

LOW CARB
midnight
Snacks

Chicken Liver Pate

Spread this pate on cucumber or celery for the ultimate low carb snack or team it with the cheese cracker recipe below.

Serves: 4
Preparation time: 10 minutes

Ingredients
1 small white onion
1 clove garlic
2 tbsp butter
2 rashers bacon
1/4 lb chicken liver
2 tbsp parsley
1 tsp nutmeg
3 tbsp cider vinegar

Method
1. Finely chop the onion and garlic and soften in the butter for 3-4 minutes.
2. Finely chop the bacon and add to the pan for 3 minutes until beginning to colour.

3. Trim any white sinews off the livers then add them, as well as the parsley and nutmeg, and fry for 5-10 minutes until the livers are cooked through, season with salt and black pepper.

4. Add the vinegar for the last couple of minutes.

5. Leave to cool then blend (in batches if necessary) until smooth.

6. Keep chilled until required.

Nutritional Information

Per serving

Calories	145
Fat (g)	11
Sodium (mg)	343
Net carbohydrates (g)	3
Sugars (g)	1
Protein (g)	9

Cheesy Crackers

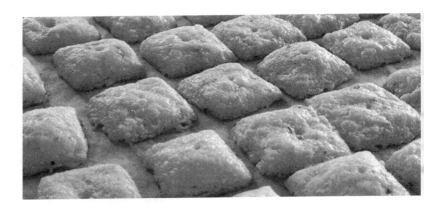

Top these crackers with the chicken liver pate, smoked mackerel mousse or just slices of cheese for a quick bite.

Serves: 4
Preparation time: 10 minutes

Ingredients
2 cups almond flour
2 medium egg whites
½ tsp rosemary
¼ tsp cayenne powder
2 tbsp parmesan cheese

Method

1. Preheat the oven to 325 degrees F.

2. Knead all the ingredients until they come together in a soft dough.

3. Lay the dough on a greased and lined baking sheet and roll out as thin as you can get it.

4. Score the dough into the size and shape of crackers you desire.

5. Bake for 8-12 minutes until browning around the edges, check the inner crackers are cooked enough and put them back in for 2-3 minutes if not.

6. Store in an airtight container until required.

Nutritional Information

Per serving

Calories	340
Fat (g)	29
Sodium (mg)	77
Net carbohydrates (g)	7
Sugars (g)	2
Protein (g)	15

Herbal Tea Ice Cream

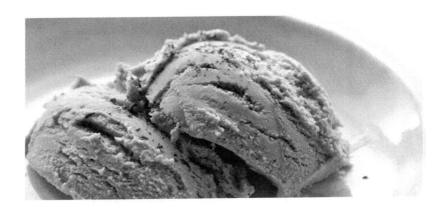

Choose any flavour of herbal tea or non-herbal tea; my favourite is a refreshing Green Tea blend, perfect for hot and sticky summer evenings. Not only is this a low carb, sweet treat but it also gives the benefits of drinking a cup of herbal tea.

Makes: 1 litre
Preparation time: 5 minutes plus 15 minutes infusing, then 24 hours freezing time

Ingredients

1 litre 2% milk
3 herbal tea bags
2 tbsp vanilla extract

Method

1. Heat the milk until it is beginning to bubble but not boiling.

2. Put the tea bags into the milk and mash them gently to release the flavours. Cover and leave to infuse for 15 minutes.

3. Strain the milk into a plastic tub and add the vanilla. Cover and freeze for 24 hours.

4. Stir the contents of the tub every 2 hours.

5. Keep frozen until ready to consume. Enjoy!

Nutritional Information

Per serving

Calories	71
Fat (g)	2
Sodium (mg)	83

Net carbohydrates (g)	8.7
Sugars (g)	5
Protein (g)	6

Zucchini Fries and Tzatziki

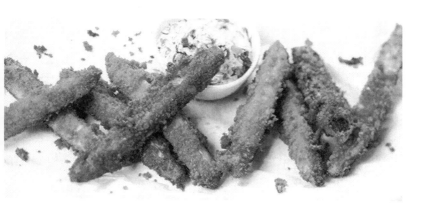

This refreshing Greek dip matches perfectly with the spiciness of the oven roasted 'fries'. Make in advance and have on hand for an emergency snack.

Serves: 4
Preparation time: 5 minutes

Ingredients
2 medium courgettes
2 tsp hot chilli powder
1/3 cup parmesan cheese
Olive oil
½ cucumber
1 clove garlic

1 cup plain Greek yogurt

2 tbsp dried parsley

Method

1. Preheat the oven to 425 degrees F.

2. Cut the courgettes into strips and dry on kitchen paper to prevent the batter going soggy.

3. Finely grate the parmesan and mix with the chilli.

4. Toss the courgettes in a little oil then coat them in the cheese mix.

5. Roast for 15-20 minutes until golden brown.

6. Grate the cucumber and squeeze out as much as possible moisture using kitchen paper.

7. Finely chop the garlic and mix well through the yogurt along with the parsley.

8. Serve immediately or keep chilled until required.

Nutritional Information
Per serving

Calories	134
Fat (g)	5.7
Sodium (mg)	287.4
Net carbohydrates (g)	5.8
Sugars (g)	1.6
Protein (g)	14

Vanilla Cheesecake

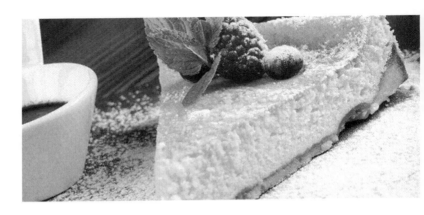

A low carb dessert perfect to enjoy at the end of a long, hard day. You can use any fruit as an accompaniment to this cake, raspberries are a good low carb option, a half cup serving is only 7 carbs.

Serves: 16
Preparation time: 10 minutes

Ingredients
100g pecans
100g ground almonds
60g butter
680g soft cream cheese
4 medium eggs

3 tbsp vanilla extract
60ml double cream
½ cup Splenda granular

Method

1. Preheat the oven to 390 degrees F.

2. Finely crush the pecans, use a food processor to speed this stage up.

3. Melt the butter in a pan and add the pecans and almonds, stir until well combined.

4. Grease a 23cm round springform baking tin and cover the bottom with the base, packing it down and into the corners well.

5. Beat together the cheese, eggs, vanilla, cream and sweetener then top the base with it.

6. As soon as the cheesecake goes into the oven, turn the temperature down to 250 degrees F and bake for 60-90 minutes, until browning on top and set.

7. Keep chilled until required.

Nutritional Information

Per serving

Calories	240
Fat (g)	22.8
Sodium (mg)	155.6
Net carbohydrates (g)	3.2
Sugars (g)	0.7
Protein (g)	6.8

Snack Sausage Rolls

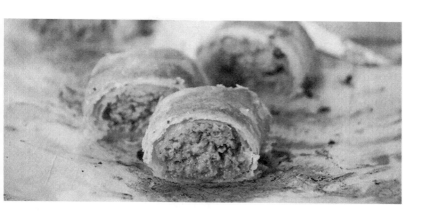

Makes 12
Preparation time: 45 minutes

Ingredients
1 garlic clove
½ cup almond flour
2 tsp oregano
½ tsp cream of tartar
1 tsp baking soda
1 tsp salt
3 large egg whites
1 large egg
½ tbsp olive oil
½ cup coconut flour

350g good quality sausage meat
1 large egg yolk

Method
1. Finely chop the garlic.
2. Place all the dry ingredients (except the coconut flour) into a bowl.
3. Whisk the egg whites, egg and oil together and add a cup of hot water. Mix into the dry mixture until fully combined.
4. Gradually add the coconut flour until it is a smooth, non-sticky dough. Chill for 30 minutes.
5. Divide the sausage meat into 12 equal portions, season well with salt and black pepper and shape into mini sausages. Chill.
6. Preheat the oven to 350 degrees F.
7. Divide the dough into 12 equal sized pieces and, using wet hands, roll out into a rectangle large enough to wrap your sausages in.
8. Wrap each sausage in the pastry rectangles and place on a greased and lined baking sheet.
9. Beat the yolk and glaze the rolls. Bake for 40 minutes until golden brown.

10. Keep chilled until required.

Nutritional Information
Per sausage roll

Calories	173
Fat (g)	11
Sodium (mg)	506
Net carbohydrates (g)	7
Sugars (g)	1
Protein (g)	11

Chicken in Yogurt and Mango Sauce

A curry style supper dish that is light enough to eat right before bed for those last minute munchies. Cooking the chicken in yogurt keeps it incredibly moist.

Serves: 4
Preparation time: 15 minutes

Ingredients
4 chicken breasts
1 small red onion
¼ cup mango
¼ plain yogurt
1 tsp ground ginger

Method
1. Preheat the oven to 350 degrees F.
2. Dice the chicken into evenly sized pieces and fry in a little olive oil until browned all over.
3. Dice the onion and mango and add to the pan with the ginger for 3 minutes.

4. Pour the yogurt in, season with salt and black pepper and stir until combined then transfer into a roasting dish and bake for 25-30 minutes until the chicken is cooked through.

5. Serve immediately or chill until required.

Nutritional Information
Per serving

Calories	296
Fat (g)	6
Sodium (mg)	129
Net carbohydrates (g)	3
Sugars (g)	2
Protein (g)	54

Conclusion

This book is packed full of delicious and nutritious recipes, it is your one stop guide to low carb snacks. While I can't guarantee weight loss, I certainly hope these recipes aid you on your quest to be your perfect weight.

Good luck on your journey!!

Printed in Great Britain
by Amazon